Platelet Transfusion

Platelet Transfusion

Edited by

T.A. Lister and J.S. Malpas

**Department of Medical Oncology
St Bartholomew's Hospital
London**

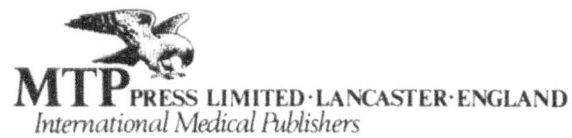

MTP **PRESS LIMITED·LANCASTER·ENGLAND**
International Medical Publishers

Published by

MTP Press Limited
Falcon House
Cable Street
Lancaster, England

British Library Cataloguing in Publication Data

International Symposium on Platelet Transfusion,
   London, 1978
   Platelet transfusion.
   1.   Blood – Transfusion – Congresses
   2.   Blood platelets – Congresses
   I.   Title   II.   Lister, T A
   III.   Malpas, J S
   615'.65   RM171
ISBN-13: 978-0-85200-248-3   e-ISBN-13: 978-94-009-8695-4

DOI: 10.1007/ 978-94-009-8695-4

Phototypesetting by Rainbow Graphics, Liverpool

4

Contents

5

List of Contributors

T. E. Cleghorn, MD, FRCP, Director, North London Blood Transfusion Centre, Edgware, Middx.

J. M. Ford, MRCP, Research Fellow and Hon. Senior Registrar, Imperial Cancer Research Fund Department of Medical Oncology, St Bartholomew's Hospital, London, EC1

Douglas W. Huestis, MD, Proffessor of Pathology, University of Arizona College of Medicine, Tucson, Arizona, USA

T. A. Lister, MD, MRCP, Senior Lecturer and Hon. Consultant Physician, Imperial Cancer Research Fund Department of Medical Oncology, St Bartholomew's Hospital, London, EC1

J. S. Malpas, DPhil, FRCP, Director, Imperial Cancer Research Fund Department of Medical Oncology, St Bartholomew's Hospital, London, EC1

Kenneth B. McCredie, MD, Associate Professor of Medicine, Department of Developmental Therapeutics, The University of Texas Cancer Center, Texas Medical Center, Houston, Texas, USA

Marion M. Roberts, FRCAP, Membrane Immunology Laboratory, Imperial Cancer Research Fund, Lincoln's Inn Fields, London, WC2

Introduction

Platelet transfusion has become an integral part of the management of disseminated malignant disease and its role in preventing or controlling haemorrhage due to thrombocytopenia is now without dispute.

This monograph contains articles presented at an International Symposium on Platelet Transfusion held in London in July 1978. It is hoped that they provide an up-to-date review of the preparation and laboratory function of platelet concentrates in addition to practical advice towards developing an intelligent approach towards their administration.

T.A. Lister
J.S. Malpas

1
Platelet Collection and Quality Control

D. Huestis

In this chapter I would like to discuss platelet collection techniques and quality control; the more clinical aspects will be covered by other contributors. In the first place it would be preferable to look at platelets from the point of view of the physician using them – what he needs to know so that his use of platelets will be intelligent and directed by background knowledge of where platelets are found, how they are harvested and stored, and the clinical realities of platelet transfusion.

The platelets we transfuse tomorrow walk the streets today. Intelligent donor recruitment and public information campaigns about blood donation, and about new systems of blood donation that are not yet familiar to the general public, need to be broadcast and developed, but are not really a subject of discussion for this meeting.

HISTORICAL REVIEW

I shall start with an historical perspective on the evolution of platelet transfusion.

When I looked into Keyne's book[1], my favourite reference for the history of blood transfusion, I did not find any mention of platelet transfusion, nor does the word 'platelet' appear in the index. The only pertinent reference is to the use of direct unmodified blood in clinical bleeding problems. In both the 1951 and 1956 editions of his book, Mollison[2] refers only briefly to platelet transfusion, and most of this again concerns the use of fresh blood in bleeding problems, although in the 1956 edition there is mention of survival studies on platelets transfused in whole blood.

Platelet transfusion proper appears in Mollison's 1961 edition, and in the American Association of Blood Banks Technical Manual[3], where the statement occurs that for the transfusion of platelets, the best method is still direct transfusion with syringes, preferably from donors with polycythaemia.

The first stage of platelet transfusion was the direct transfusion of unmodified blood, either artery-to-vein in the earlier days, or later, less heroic systems of vein-to-vein transfusion. As late as 1960, the semi-direct method, using multiple syringes of unmodified or little modified whole blood was considered best.

The next stage, in the 1950s, emphasized the use of siliconized glass bottles. Plastic bag systems were in their infancy then, but the techniques of differential centrifugation to separate platelet-rich plasma from whole blood, then platelets from platelet-rich plasma, were developed at that time. It was considered essential to submit the freshly-collected blood to rapid chilling, even at times drawing the blood into pre-chilled containers, so that there would be absolutely minimal maintenance of blood at higher temperatures. This was on the premise that the platelet was a very delicate little particle, and if not chilled immediately it was bound to undergo a rapid demise. This, as we now know, was not the best way to do things, but surprisingly enough it worked on many occasions.

It was noticed that when platelets were collected like this, clumping tended to occur, and that collection in full EDTA prevented clumping, so EDTA was initially recommended as an anticoagulant for platelets. At this stage there was little or no mention of storage. If the platelet was so fragile that it had to be collected and chilled immediately, then of course it could not be stored for very long. Cronkite and Jackson's review[4], stated that siliconized syringes were still the best method of transfusing platelets, preferably from polycythaemic donors.

The third stage, in the 1960s saw the gradual abandonment of glass bottles and the faster abandonment of EDTA. Plastic blood-bag systems were by that time well worked out, although by no means in widespread use until the later 1960s. A slight lowering of pH by the addition of extra ACD decreased platelet clumping and improved post-transfusion survival. There was still uncertainty about storage. Most people considered that storage was possible, but not desirable. I am not entirely sure that that is wrong. In our own textbook[5], we said platelets could be kept for about 24 hours, but it was certainly better to transfuse them immediately.

12

There was, however, at this time, a great escalation in clinical usage, which began to make it impractical to collect platelets only on direct order for specific patients, so that changes had to be made to the collection system. Simultaneously came the early development of plateletpheresis, including multiple bag plateletpheresis and the appearance of the cell separator, with the aim of collecting large amounts of platelets from a single normal donor.

In the 1970s, concurrent with the explosive acceleration of the clinical usage of platelets, we saw great improvements in platelet storage, and the potential to store viable platelets for two or three days. The controversy over storage systems, still not entirely resolved, has been quite acrimonious at times, with the 4°C camp vying against the 22°C camp. Concurrent with the rapid increase in platelet transfusion in leukaemic patients, came an awareness of the clinically refractory state, in which patients fail to respond to platelet transfusions, and of the importance of histocompatibility in platelet transfusions.

Plateletpheresis has also rapidly developed in the past few years, with the use of selected platelet donors, and concurrent with that the evolution of techniques for the freezing and thawing of platelets. However, these techniques are as yet not standardized and should still be considered experimental.

A five-year summary of American National Red Cross[6] usage of components, completed in 1975, shows the increase in the issuance of platelet preparations over that period of time. An extraordinarily rapid rise parallels the rise in the usage of blood components as opposed to whole blood.

After these stages of development, systems of platelet collection and separation, in the US at least, became fixed and standardized, almost like the Law of the Medes and the Persians.

CURRENT SYSTEMS OF COLLECTION AND SEPARATION OF PLATELETS

1. Whole blood in a multiple plastic bag system

The basic concept is to collect whole blood into three or four integrally connected plastic containers allowing the aseptic separation of components by sequential centrifugation steps. Whole blood is

13

collected in the primary bag, then a soft centrifugation leaves red blood cells in the primary bag and allows the expression of platelet-rich plasma into a satellite bag. Following removal of the primary container, centrifugation of the platelet-rich plasma gives platelet-poor plasma in one satellite bag and a platelet concentrate in another.

Using a four-bag system and a similar procedure, one can separate the red blood cells and platelet concentrate, then subject the platelet-poor plasma to the rapid freeze and slow thaw that gives cryo-precipitated anti-haemophilic factor and cryoprecipitate-poor plasma. This makes maximal use out of a single blood donation to produce multiple components.

2. Platelet storage

Although it is best to transfuse platelets immediately after separation, it is not always logistically possible to do so. Levin and Freireich[7] showed poor platelet increments after transfusion of stored platelet-rich plasma, stored for 24 and 48 hours, compared with unstored fresh platelets.

Murphy and Gardner[8] found rather poor post-transfusion survival of platelets stored for 8 hours and 18 hours, at both 4 °C and 22 °C, with less effectiveness at the lower temperature.

Recent work sheds some light on the dispute between the advocates of 4 °C and 22 °C storage. Filip and Aster[9] found no difference in post-transfusion survival at 4 hours and 72 hours except in the case of platelets kept for 72 hours at 4°C, where recovery was significantly impaired. The shortening of bleeding time, as a measure of haemostatic effectiveness, was studied in transfused platelets stored in the same set of circumstances. Once again, the platelets stored at 4°C for 72 hours were not as effective. None of the other results were significantly different from each other.

From this, Filip and Aster concluded that 4°C storage is not desirable for more than 24 hours, but that within the first 24 hours it does not make much difference whether the platelets are stored at 4°C or at 22°C. However, if they are to be stored for longer than that, the 22°C system should be used.

One thread of truth running through the whole story of platelet transfusion from the earliest days is worth emphasizing because it is often forgotten. There is a great scatter of results in all different circumstances. We can transfuse platelets that have been subjected to quite a variety of collection and storage procedures and still achieve effective platelet transfusion. When we collected platelets and spun them in centrifuge cups packed with ice, a procedure we now know to be undesirable, many of the patients stopped bleeding. This is something that we have to keep in mind.

Based on many studies of the kind cited, one can say that cold-stored platelets do not survive as well in the recipient after transfusion, but they have the advantage of being somewhat stickier than platelets collected and stored at higher temperatures. Consequently they seem to have a better immediate effect in the bleeding thrombocytopenic patient. Thus, for *immediate* effect platelets stored in the cold may be better if they are not stored for more than 24 hours, whereas if the concern is more for prophylactic use in thrombocytopenic patients who are not immediately bleeding, then the platelets stored at room temperature could be considered better. If it were feasible to maintain both systems, this might be best. However, it is not really practical to do things that way, and a room temperature system appears to offer the most advantages.

To summarize the present empirical system of platelet preparation and storage:

1. Fresh whole blood is collected and is not subjected to chilling.
2. The soft centrifugation procedure is carried out at 20°C at approximately $1740\,g$ for a few minutes (3 minutes) to separate the red cells from the platelet-rich plasma.
3. Following this, the separated platelet-rich plasma is given a higher g-force centrifugation, still at 20°C, in order to separate platelets from plasma.

(Most centres in the US do not recombine the platelet-poor plasma with the red cells, but such an option can be used to produce a modified whole blood, if that is what is wanted. Consequently the system has considerable flexibility.)

4. If the platelet concentrate is to be stored at 4°C, then a small amount of plasma is left on the platelets which are allowed to remain *undisturbed* for one hour at 22°C. Undisturbed means no labelling or handling at all. Alternatively, the platelets may be rotated *gently*. This prevents them from sticking together and

15

forming aggregates. After this period they may be put in the refrigerator at 4°C and agitation is not required. Storage should probably be limited to 24 hours. Shipment is relatively easy because they can be placed in wet ice, in boxes, and shipped almost anywhere, since 4°C is relatively easy to maintain.

5. For storage at 22°C, more plasma (50–70 ml) must be left on the platelets. This is to maintain the platelet pH. During storage, they require gentle continuous agitation and adequate ventilation. This too apparently helps to maintain the pH and the respiration of the platelets. This may be an important consideration in platelets collected by plateletpheresis where a large volume of concentrate may be kept in a small plastic bag and may not then achieve adequate ventilation. (See Katz[10])

The 72-hour storage seems to be quite reasonable for platelets that are prepared and handled in this way, but what remains uncertain is the optimal shipping conditions for them. In my own area, if we were to ship without some cooling, the platelets might reach ambient temperatures of over 100°F which, to say the least, would be highly undesirable for their storage and function. They should certainly be protected from extremes of temperature.

3. Plateletpheresis

This brings us to plateletpheresis, the collection of platelets by techniques that enable the red cells and the plasma to be returned to the donor, so that larger numbers of platelets are obtained from fewer donors, with the added potential for being able to take platelets from a donor more frequently than the usual time interval permitted for donation of blood. These techniques are not necessarily complex. Simple multiple bag systems can be adapted from those already described, or various machines can be used, predominantly the Haemonetics machine utilizing the Latham bowl. The latter is a disposable polycarbonate centrifuge bowl in which the blood enters while the bowl is spinning, with the g-forces forcing the red cells to the outside, the plasma to the inside, and the buffy coat forming in between. As the bowl fills and the plasma separates, the plasma flows into an outside collection bag, and the buffy coat rises to the top, from where it is diverted to another collection bag. After this, the plasma and the red cells, by reversal of flow, are sent back to the donor, and the whole process is repeated. The system is a two-arm procedure. The antecubital vein in one arm is used for the primary blood donation site. The anticoagulant joins the donor blood as it enters the tubing. The return is to the donor's other arm, preferably in a forearm or hand vein, so that the donor can move one hand. With this procedure, in a donation period of 2 hours or less, the number of platelets collected would be equivalent to anywhere from 10 to 12 or more conventional platelet concentrates.

Practising physicians are not generally label-oriented, but they are advised to read the labels of the blood products they use, to obtain essential information. In plateletpheresis, for example, the number of platelets usually obtained is 6 or 7×10^{11}, equivalent to about 10 or so conventional platelet concentrates. The rest of the information is cautionary details concerning the laboratory tests and the actual administration. This is important, because when platelet concentrates are sent to hospitals the hospital blood bank is likely to put them immediately in the refrigerator, and it is better not to do so. Since most pheresis collections, are collected from a specific donor for a specific patient, we always prefer that they be given immediately rather than stored. The less the storage, the better the clinical results. We have seen instances in which the patients were apparently refractory because they were getting for the most part 3-day-old platelet concentrates stored at 4°C, and the refractoriness was more apparent than real.

When platelets are collected from a patient's relative, a brother, a sister, or a parent, there is a temptation to use the same donor again the next day. This can be done, but the bone marrow does not replenish platelets as fast as one would like, and the donor can experience a considerable fall in platelet count in sequential pheresis.

The fall in platelet count is roughly proportional to the donor's original platelet count. If he has an initial count of $500 \times 10^9/1$, after one plateletpheresis his count will be less than $300 \times 10^9/1$, and if he is pheresed again the very next day he will probably go down to around $200 \times 10^9/1$ and so on. The fall in platelet count has to be watched.

It is possible, by slightly modifying the procedure, to minimise loss of red cells in plateletpheresis, and this is an important consideration for the donor subjected to repeated plateletpheresis. Here is a system that we originally used. If the buffy coat is collected for $2\frac{1}{2}$ minutes from the time the platelet ring approaches the centre of the bowl, the total platelet yield is 7×10^{11}. But, if that is done, the donor loses 82 ml

17

packed red cells. However, if the collection time for each cycle was reduced from 2½ minutes to 1½ minutes, the yield was 6.3 as against 7 but we halved the loss of red cells. Some physicians are concerned about the number of red cells in units of platelets, but removal of red cells by centrifugation usually removes about 20% of the platelets as well, and I have generally felt that this is not warranted under most circumstances. When it is warranted, it can be done, just as one can under other circumstances remove the excess plasma.

Recruitment

Recruitment of donors for plateletpheresis is by no means easy, because the donor must sacrifice at least 2 hours, which is particularly difficult for the non-related donors who are needed for patients who do not have family members available. Recruitment and co-ordination even in a small service takes considerable time and effort, and requires most of one person's time. It is no easy job. Indeed, dealing with family members is often as difficult as co-ordinating unrelated donors, or even more so.

Effect of aspirin

When donors are recruited for plateletpheresis the aspirin effect should be borne in mind. If the patient has no platelets and the donor took aspirin the day before, his platelets would probably be useless for that particular patient. Aspirinated platelets may fail to correct the bleeding time in thrombocytopenic patients.

4. Quality control

Certainly careful collection is very important. In particular, atraumatic venepuncture should be aimed for. Also, careful agitation of the container during the collection of the blood for platelet concentrates must always be observed, and the duration of collection watched. These influence the usefulness of the platelets so obtained.

Fresher platelet concentrates are preferred, particularly with apparently refractory patients. This is an extremely important concept. The clinical decision as to the type of patient who will or will not respond to platelet concentrates is probably the most important consideration of all, and the proper handling of platelets sent from a community blood centre to a hospital is likewise extremely important.

In the US we have set a minimum requirement of 5.5×10^{10} platelets per regular concentrate, which is supposed to be demonstrable in at least three-quarters of platelet concentrates tested for quality control.

Other important considerations are the amount of plasma, the storage temperature, the size of the bag in relation to the amount of plasma[10] and ventilation. The pH of the collected platelets must not descend below 6.0, and perhaps most important of all is the clinical rather than the laboratory evaluation of the outcome of the transfusions. We will be wise to remember that the most relevant factor about platelet transfusion is whether it stops bleeding.

References

1. Keynes, G. L. (1949). *Blood Transfusion.* (Bristol: John Wright)
2. Mollison, P. L. (1956). *Blood Transfusion in Clinical Medicine.* (Oxford: Oxford University Press)
3. American Association of Blood Banks' Technical Manual. (1960)
4. Cronkite and Jackson. (1959). In L. M. Tocantins (ed.) *Progress in Haematology,* Vol. 2. (New York: Grune and Stratton)
5. Huestis, D. W., Bove, J. R. and Busch, S. (1969). *Practical Blood Transfusion.* (Boston: Little, Brown and Co.)
6. American National Red Cross Usage of Components. (1975)
7. Levin, R. H. and Freireich, E. J. (1964). Effect of storage up to 48 hours on response to transfusions of platelet rich plasma. *Transfusion,* **4,** 251
8. Murphy, S. and Gardner, F. H. (1969). Platelet preservation. Effect of storage temperature on maintenance of platelet viability-deleterious effect on refrigerated storage. *New Engl. J. Med.,* **280,** 1094
9. Filip, D. J. and Aster, R. H. (1978). Relative hemostatic effectiveness of human platelets stored at 4 degrees and 22 degrees centigrade. *J. Lab. Clin. Med.,* **91,** 618
10. Katz, A., Houx, J. and Ewald, L. (1978). Storage of platelets prepared by discontinuous flow centrifugation. *Transfusion,* **18,** 220

2
Platelet Collection at Edgware
T.E. Cleghorn

During the second half of 1967, the preparation of cryoprecipitate was introduced at Edgware and within a matter of weeks more than 1000 units per week were being produced. This level of production was maintained until last year when demand fell as a result of the increasing availability of factor VIII concentrates. Also in 1967 I was advised that an explosive demand for platelet concentrates, similar to that for cryoprecipitate was likely to materialize within the next 2 years. A series of consultations and studies followed and in mid-1969 the decision was taken, with some trepidation, to operate an on-call platelet bank rather than to scale-up the *ad hoc* supply arrangements against demand which had operated hitherto. At that time, technology was far from clear and development of our systems followed some experimental work and rather more guess work. Finance was an overriding consideration and we began with the intention, if at all possible, to utilise the same donation for platelet preparation as for cryoprecipitate production. This meant that we had to rule out techniques which involved additional acid–citrate–dextrose (ACD), as otherwise factor VIII yields would suffer. This led in turn to a need to avoid platelet concentration against foreign surfaces with consequent aggregation in the absence of increased acidity.

A series of experiments showed that platelets could be separated in apparently normal condition from buffy coats, even when the latter had been prepared by hard centrifugation of the whole blood donation. This separation was readily effected by transferring the buffy coat and some plasma to another satellite pack, gently resuspending the cells, and then subjecting them to a slow spin when white cells and erythrocytes were readily deposited, leaving quite

21

remarkably clean platelet-rich plasma as supernatant. It was also found convenient to pool buffy coats from five donations thus filling to capacity the standard transfer pack adopted and allowing a clean separation by centrifugation. Pooling and transfer operations were carried out in a Microflow cabinet.

From this experimentation, standard production procedures were developed and since 1969 we have issued just under 40 000 of these packs to the hospitals which we serve.

Apart from the above considerations, a number of other options were decided in 1969. First we standardized on Fenwal packs which seemed to be best suited to the procedures adopted and we have had no reason to regret this decision. Second, we opted for room temperature preparation and storage. This fitted in well with the cryoprecipitation and was economical of transport and centrifuge time. By so doing, however, we denied ourselves the option of platelet preparation from overnight blood and increased the pressures in the components laboratory by the necessity to prepare platelets from freshly collected blood before it was refrigerated. I have never been happy about the term room-temperature, which may be more meaningful in air-conditioned environments, but certainly embraces a pretty wide range of temperatures in United Kingdom. What we do is to transport the blood donations from donor clinic to components laboratory in open containers without refrigeration and then carry out the two centrifugations at stabilized 20°C. Storage of the concentrates is also stabilized at this temperature.

A third decision taken was to keep the platelets in suspension by constant agitation during storage. The evidence to support this was not all that strong in 1969, but it is now standard practice. We use an orbital incubator with a slow horizontal circular movement. This is not particularly effective and we are looking for something better although currently, there is no problem as bank storage is only transient while demand is so high.

The current standard procedure for platelet collection is summarized in Figures 1 and 2. The donation is spun hard, most of the plasma is transferred to one satellite, the buffy coat with some plasma is transferred to a second satellite and detached. Five buffy coats are then pooled in a transfer pack, spun slowly and then the platelet rich plasma is transferred to a second transfer pack, sealed and labelled. Only donations of the same ABO groups are used in any one pool and Rh type is ignored unless there are clinical indications for a Rhesus

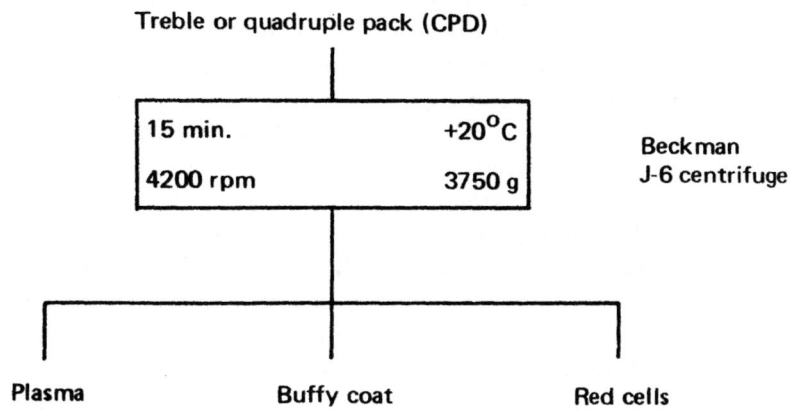

Figure 1 Preparation of platelet rich plasma (Stage II)

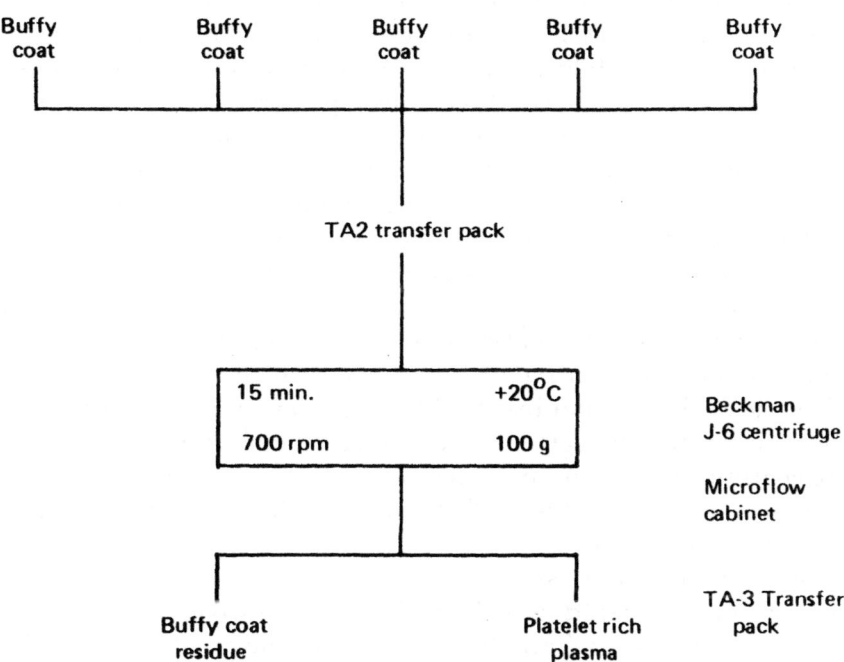

Figure 2 Preparation of platelet-rich plasma (Stage I)

negative preparation. In such circumstances when a sufficient number of Rhesus negative donors cannot be assembled in time, platelets from Rhesus positive donors are supplied with the advice that prophylactic anti-D immunoglobulin should be given. While the initial spin and transfers are in progress, ABO and Rh confirmation, syphilis screening and rapid Hepatest procedures are put in hand. However, since hepatitis high-risk donors are not used for component preparation, except in times of great demand or shortage, syphilis is rarely seen and donors of known groups are used. (Newly enrolled donors are placed in the hepatitis high-risk category for their first donation and tested for hepatitis B surface antigen by solid-phase RIA as well as by Hepatest.) Completion of the preparation proceeds ahead of screening results being received. Issue, of course, is not allowed until laboratory clearance has been given.

The main preparative operation is restricted to the 5 weekdays with cover for the weekend coming from the bank. This makes Friday a pretty hectic day. Smaller, selective preparative operations are mounted during weekends which extend into national holidays. The only variation on this standard procedure is in respect of specific requests for small children when five donor units would be wasteful and in such cases a pack of three units is prepared. Specific measures for donor selection are not possible when working on this scale but those confessing to aspirin taking are excluded. Otherwise, all donors whose blood is suitable for routine hospital issue are included.

Attention has been drawn on many occasions to the bacteriological hazards of room temperature storage which must, *ipso facto*, be higher than those at 4°C. The importance of skin cleansing prior to venesection for blood donation has been stressed, and it is only at this stage in closed-system blood processing, that the system is open to airborne or skin contaminants. There are conflicting accounts in the literature as to the degree of contamination encountered in platelet concentrates stored at room temperature. This variation may be technical and a function of the size of the inoculum which is submitted to culture.

In designing our system, we were acutely aware of this bacteriological hazard and appreciated that it would not be acceptable in America or Canada. Initially, we subjected every pooled pack to culture and requested donor-line segments from users. Once we had developed our sampling and culture techniques – and plastic blood packs are by no means easy to manipulate in microbiological techniques without accidental contamination – we found that the contamination rate was extremely low and we now culture a random

24

10% sample. Approximate figures for the incidence of contamination are shown in Table 1. In this the figures for production are presented in terms of packs of five donor units, and are not particularly accurate. The figures for contamination are lower than most of those found in the literature and this is almost certainly due to the small size of the inoculum used for culture. The technique which we use currently is seen in Table 2 and it will be noted that the inoculum is extremely small in relation to the size of the pack.

Table 1 Incidence of bacterial contamination of platelet concentrates

| | | | *Number positive* | |
	Approx. number produced	*Approx.* number tested	*Probable* real contamination	*Probable* sampling contamination
1973	?	3000	2	8
1974	5000	5000	1	1
1975	6000	1000	0	0
1976	7000	2300	1*	1
1977	8500	5000	0	2
1978 (to June)	5000	500	0	0

* Associated with open-system pack connectors

Note: 1. Most positives are Gram positive cocci.
2. 673 cell separator samples tested to date were negative.

Table 2 Screening for bacteriological contamination of platelet concentrates

Sampling

1. Clean the bleed line portion to be sample in 70% ethanol
2. Snip the end off with flame-sterilized scissors
3. Squeeze out drop of sample onto plate

Incubation

1. 30°C (blood agar plate)
2. 25°C (nutrient agar plate)

These tests must of necessity be only of retrospective value except for preparations which have been banked for more than 16–18 hours when gross contamination could be expected to be detectable. The hospital segments would provide the best indicator of the microbiological status of our product. We never got more than 10% of these back and never had any convincing evidence of contamination – they are even more tricky to handle than are packs and melt if flamed with spirit.

With consistently negative results, the hospitals soon lost interest in returning segments and we seldom see any now. I shall return to this topic when discussing future developments.

Other quality control of the product comprises regular counting of random samples and reveals interesting variations between centrifuges. Also, more sporadic measurements of pH, aggregation and clot retraction. Microscopical inspection for white and red cell contamination will be introduced shortly.

The counting reveals pretty wide variations between packs, with an average content of about 1.2×10^{11} platelets per pack with a standard deviation of 0.3. This is low compared with calculated yields and with those found with classical methods of preparation. Indices of function have always been within normal limits and there has been no feed-back from hospitals to suggest that the preparations are not clinically effective.

About 10% of our production comes from donors undergoing plasmapheresis. The majority of these donate for specific immunoglobulin production – anti-HBs, anti-HZ, anti-measles, anti-rubella in the 'naturally occurring' group and anti-tetanus, anti-A and anti-B, and anti-rabies in those specifically immunized or boosted. Donors of anti-D are not used because the loss of antibody in the suspending plasma would be unacceptably high.

During the last year, we have installed and are now operating a Haemonetics cell separator. At full load, this is calculated to do four runs a day, 5 days a week and each run produces roughly the equivalent of two of our standard packs of platelets. Currently, it averages 16 runs a week and is making a significant contribution to production.

Before discussing future trends and developments, it may be interesting to consider the financial aspects of production from our three sources of material. In order to produce 3.0×10^{11} platelets, the plastic pack and ancillary costs in our hands are as follows: single donor units by classical technique £10; Edgware pools £24; Haemonetics £30. The relatively high cost of the Edgware pools has to be seen in the context of the simultaneous yield of cryoprecipitate or fresh frozen plasma.

In summary, we are making a clinically acceptable product in quantities adequate to meet current hospital demand. Where do we go from here?

First, the number of units issued per year has increased steadily since 1969, with only a brief drop between 1973 and 1975. Two thousand donor units were issued in 1969 compared with a predicted number (based on the first 6 months of the year) of 4700 in 1978. In our earlier years, some 15% of production was unused, last year 10%, the first 5 months of 1978, 8%, in June 1978, 3% and July nil. This may represent seasonal variation, but as absolute figures are rising, it is much more likely due to genuine expansion of demand, and is most probably related to the increase in marrow grafting operations.

It is necessary, therefore, to consider how we can predict the level of demand in the future, and then how we can meet it. Production of platelet concentrates by American Red Cross Blood Centres rose from 81 125 in 1969 to 902 896 in 1976 – an eleven-fold increase which is of the same order as our 15-fold increase in issues in the same period.

If the figure of 902 896 really represents satisfaction of demand, then we have to admit to commitment by Edgware in 1978, of some 6% of total United States Red Cross production! If we are to confine platelet production to single shift processing of fresh blood, then clearly we have reached our limit in this direction as far as routine donation is concerned, unless we are prepared to bleed into surplus. While this would admittedly appeal to users of factor VIII and of albumin, I have never accepted that donated red cells can properly be discarded unused, as our German and Swiss colleagues have done. Admittedly they now dispose of some surplus to New York, but I do not doubt that this balance of payments deficit will also soon be corrected.

We must, therefore, examine two other possibilities. First, to increase the yield of platelets harvested per donation and/or second, to expand our collection by some form of platelet-pheresis.

In regard to the first alternative, there is little doubt that we could almost double the absolute number of platelets which we extract from fresh donations by adopting the classical method of production. Without somewhat complicated manoeuvres in a pretty expansive quadruple pack system, however, we would end up with one third of our blood as concentrated cells. Not only would we incur the wrath of most surgeons and anaesthetists, but also pressure on albumin supply would be renewed, and the whole system would go out of balance. An alternative would be to use the classical system, but take platelets from a smaller volume of platelet-rich plasma. This would however, necessitate an extensive pooling operation either at Edgware or in hospital. Admittedly, we do such now, but we are under pressure from the medicines inspectorate, either to conduct such operations in white-area (operating theatre) conditions, or to discontinue them. The problems of sterilizing the exterior of blood packs have not been solved and it looks as if pooling operations are out. Perhaps one day the inspectors will have time to watch their television sets and see blood packs hanging up in operating theatres to the dismay of none.

The alternative of pooling single platelet units in hospitals is certainly feasible, but does add one more irritating task to our load. I am in no doubt that we could do it better in the Centre.

Another approach is to increase production by cell separator and this has many attractions. There is incontravertible evidence that the wider the exposure to platelets from different donors, the higher is the probability that platelet antibodies will develop. Once developed, then matched platelet transfusion will be obligatory except perhaps when bleeding has to be controlled and maintenance levels are a thing of the future.

Given the clinical desirability of such a course of action, I have little doubt that the necessary finance would be forthcoming with the usual benevolent reluctance of the powers that be. There are two additional considerations. First we can recruit the necessary donors in sufficient numbers? My view and experience is that we can, provided that we can provide good accommodation with adequate staffing to avoid waiting. The second consideration is, are we sure that we need platelets in the quantities envisaged? If we are, and clinicians must be asked to review their activities in critical fashion, then we will go ahead with cell separation. It is, however, more than one small step which is needed to convert users from prescribing by the five-donor pack – one, two or three – to specification of an absolute number of platelets per kilogramme for a given patient.

3
Effectiveness of Platelet Transfusion and Laboratory Function of Platelets
M. Roberts

INTRODUCTION

Platelet concentration may be obtained either by the pooling of platelet rich plasma from singly collected units of whole blood or by the separation of whole blood in a flow system. At St Bartholomew's Hospital both sources are used to obtain platelets for supply to patients with acute leukaemia. This study investigated the clinical effectiveness and laboratory characteristics of platelets obtained from the Haemonetics cell separator.

YIELDS

Six units of National Blood Transfusion Service platelet concentrate were given as a single transfusion and contained a mean of 2.3×10^{11} platelets when stored and collected at $4\,^{\circ}\mathrm{C}$ or of 2.6×10^{11} platelets when stored and collected at $22\,^{\circ}\mathrm{C}$. A mean yield of 4.3×10^{11} platelets per collection was achieved with four runs of a 375 ml bowl in the Haemonetics Model 30 cell separator. Donor problems with the cell separator were rare. Acid citrate dextrose-A was used as the anticoagulant and 4% of donors had some citrate reaction. This consisted of slight paraethesia and occasionally cramps. Four per cent also had some symptoms of hypotension but these side effects often coincided. In all cases the reactions were very mild. The procedure took less than 2 hours and cross-matching was done during this time, so the platelets could be used immediately after collection. As the cell separator provides enough platelets for therapeutic transfusion from a single donor and as that donor may donate again repeatedly at

29

quite short intervals without a fall in haemoglobin, the number of donors needed is small compared to those needed for platelet concentrate transfusions. Another advantage is that a relative or a selected donor can be used. We have used a single donor eight times in 32 days and another donor seven times in 24 days without a fall in either the platelet count or the haemoglobin over this time.

DESIGN OF THE STUDY

To study the function of the platelets from the cell separator, we compared the platelets taken from the bag immediately after collection on the separator with control platelets which were taken directly from the donor's vein as the cannula needles were inserted. The control platelets were anticoagulated with the ACD in the same proportions as were used for cell separation. Thus we compared the donor's platelets before they had been processed by the cell separator with his own platelets after they had been collected. We also compared these to the platelet concentrates from the blood transfusion centre. We assessed the platelet function in both *in vitro* and *in vivo* tests.

IN VITRO TESTS

Methods

The hypotonic stress test was described by Fantl[1] and tests the actual viability of the platelets. The platelets are exposed to a hypotonic medium abruptly; they change in size and if viable return to their normal size. We found this alteration in size occurred normally in all the preparations of platelets.

Aggregation of the platelets was tested with adenosine diphosphate (ADP) and collagen as aggregating agents. Testing with both agents is necessary to distinguish between a thrombocytopathic and a thrombocytothemic abnormality. Platelet collection samples were adjusted to a constant platelet concentration by dilution with Owren's buffer.

Results

Cell separator platelets vs normal controls

We found decreased aggregation in 17 out of 41 of collected platelets: decreased aggregation being defined as loss of aggregation at the lowest concentration of ADP necessary to induce aggregation in the control. This required a substantial change in platelet response

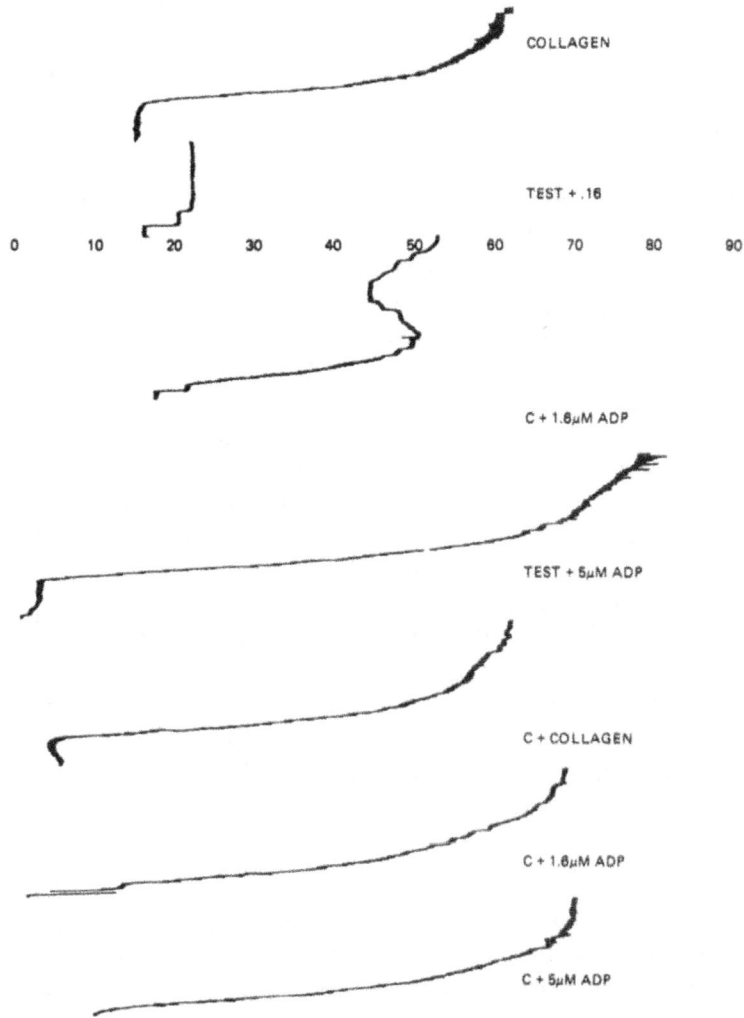

Figure 1 Platelet aggregation curves

31

Table 1 Percentage of samples achieving second degree aggregation

		n	ADP Concentration (μmol/l) 1.6	5	16.6	Collagen
CS platelets	Pre*	41	74	79	100	90
	Post†	41	54	59	71	81
CS + HES‡ platelets	Pre*	27	56	100	100	100
	Post†	27	11	42	54	90
Platelet concentrations		19		0	17	9

*   Control platelets taken from donor before separation procedure begins.

†   Platelets from the collected bag immediately after the separation.

‡   Hydroxyl Ethyl Starch used to increase yield in granulocyte donations.

because ADP concentrations used in the test were 1.6 μmol/l, 5 μmol/l and 16.6 μmol/l. There was no aggregation difference between control and collected platelets in response to collagen. Figure 1 is an example of the aggregation curves obtained. The first three curves are the control platelets from the donor before any separation procedure, using 5 and 1.6 μmol/l ADP and collagen, showing complete second degree aggregation. The test platelets after collection also aggregate at 5 μmol/l ADP, but at 1.6 they show only first degree aggregation. Table 1 shows the percentage of cell separated platelets achieving second degree aggregation at different concentrations of ADP compared to the control pre-collection platelets from the same donor. There is a decrease in platelet aggregation after collection.

Platelets obtained while collecting granulocytes for granulocyte transfusions had a much greater defect in their aggregation after collection. These platelets were collected in the presence of hydroxy ethyl starch (HES) and it is interesting to note that HES, when used as a plasma expander, has occasionally been reported to cause bleeding defects in patients.

Blood transfusion service platelets

Only 17% of platelet concentrates showed second degree aggregation with the 16.6 μmol/l concentration of ADP, and only 9% aggregated with collagen. These concentrates were usually used and tested 24 hours after collection. Some were stored at 4°C and others at 22°C. The platelet concentrates were also slighly more acidic than the cell

32

separated platelets and this is known to inhibit aggregation. Buffering the platelet concentrates to the pH of the cell separator platelets did not improve their function even after 4 hours at that pH.

Tullis pioneered the work with the cell separators and noted in his first paper[2] that ADP aggregation of the platelets was slightly decreased. The reason for this decrease in aggregation is not yet defined. Friedberg[3] has suggested that during centrifugation the platelets release their own ADP due to trauma, and so become refractory for a time to added ADP and to aggregation. Because of this, we measured the ADP levels in the donor's platelets before and after the collecting centrifugation (Table 2). There is no difference between the ADP levels in the platelets before centrifuging in the collecting system and afterwards. The ADP refractoriness, described by Friedberg, reversed in a few hours, but our separated platelets did not recover and their aggregation defect remained constant over several hours.

Table 2 ADP* levels in nmol/10^9 platelets

Sample	Pre-separation	post-separation
1	32	27
2	11	27
3	25	22
4	35	34
5	23	22
6	26	22

* ADP estimation was performed by Mr D Perrett of St Bartholomew's Hospital by high performance liquid chromatography on trichloracetic acid extracts of the platelets.

So to summarize in the *in vitro* results, we found that the hypotonic stress test, which is a crude test of viability or membrane integrity, was normal in both types of platelets tested. Aggregation induced by ADP was slightly decreased in the cell separator platelets and to a greater degree in the blood transfusion platelet concentrates.

In vivo **function**

Methods

The tests used to estimate *in vivo* function were the platelet increment and the bleeding time at one hour (Duke's method). We found that clinical effectiveness was not useful as a measure of platelet function because the indications for the platelet transfusions and the circumstances of transfusion were so variable.

Results

Figure 2 shows the increments obtained after transfusion of the platelet concentrates and the cell separator platelets. The increment is expressed for 10^{11} platelets given and per square metre of surface area of the recipient, so that the increments obtained in different patients can be compared. The mean of the increments is the same. Excluding the patients who were antibody-positive on screening reveals some difference but this is not statistically significant. The detrimental effects on the platelet increments of fever and disseminated intravascular coagulation were recognized.

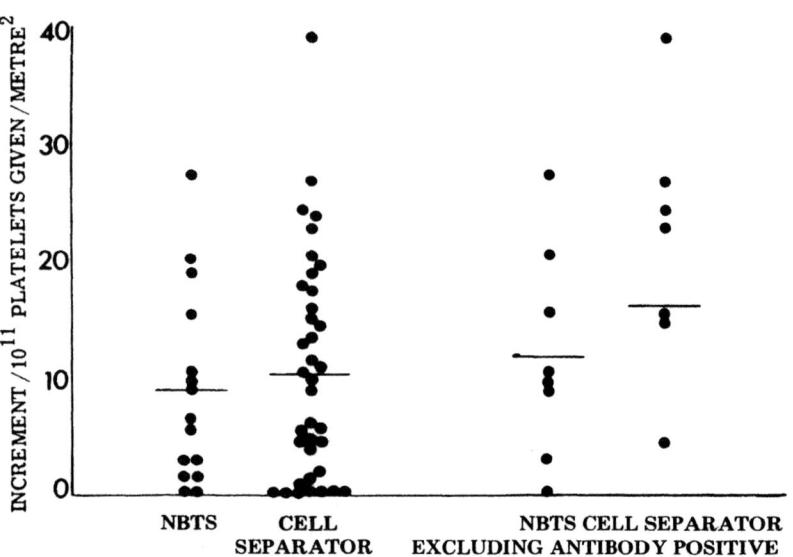

Figure 2 Increments obtained after transfusion of the platelet concentrates and the cell separator platelets

Bleeding time was assessed by Duke's method (the earprick bleeding time) because most of the patients were very thrombocytopenic and very neutropenic as well. They were all done by the same person. Bleeding time was assessed before the transfusion and then 1 hour after the transfusion, at the same time as the increment was taken, and was used as a measure of the effectiveness *in vivo* of the transfused platelets.

Figure 3 shows the reduction in bleeding time expressed as a per cent reduction compared to the increment in platelet count. The reduction in bleeding time was not related to the increment that was obtained by the platelets given. It also showed that the cell separator platelets were more effective in decreasing bleeding time than the concentrates for the same increment obtained in platelet counts.

O = Cell Separator platelets
● = NBTS Platelet concentrates

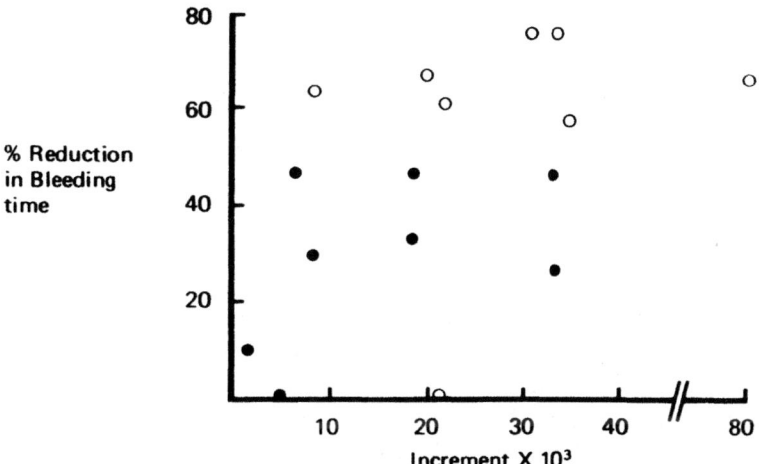

Figure 3 Percentage reduction in bleeding time as a function of the increment in platelet count

The reduction in bleeding time did not appear to be dose related, at least in the ranges of platelet dose studied, as shown in Figure 4 and for the same number of platelets given, the cell separator platelets gave the greater reduction in bleeding time than the platelet concentrates (although there are only a few cases where the number of platelets given from the cell separator were as low in numbers as those from the platelet concentrates).

Our *in vivo* studies then showed that the reduction in bleeding time was not related to the platelet dose, or to the increment obtained, but was related to the type of platelets transfused. The reduction in bleeding time was greater after cell separator platelets than it was after the platelet concentrate transfusions.

35

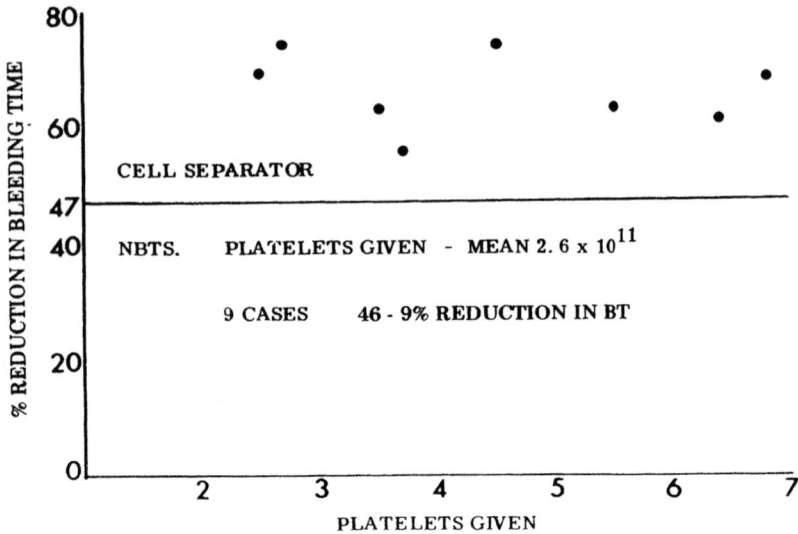

Figure 4 Percentage reduction in bleeding time as a function of platelet dose

Comment

Very little has been reported of functional assessment of platelets obtained from the cell separators. Tullis originally found a mean reduction in bleeding time of 80% but this was only in eight transfusions. Koepke[4] has labelled cell separator collected autologous platelets with chromium-51 and transfused them back into the normal volunteers from whom they were taken, and found that their survival was normal.

Our study has confirmed that, although *in vitro* aggregation tests show some defect in the platelets following collection, the clinical experience of the effectiveness of the platelets transfused from the Haemonetics cell separator is well justified, and bleeding times have shown that these platelets are indeed quite functional and effective. Added to this effectiveness are the other advantages of platelets from the cell separator, such as the ease and the rapidity of collection, and the ability to select a low number of donors, thus reducing the likelihood of any sensitization.

References

1. Fantl, P. (1968). Osmotic stability of blood platelets. *J. Physiol.*, **198**, 1
2. Tullis, J. L., Eberle, W. G., Baudanza, P. and Tinch, R. (1968). Plateletpheresis – description of a new technique. *Transfusion*, **8**, 154
3. Friedberg, N. M. and Zucher, M. B. (1972). ADP as the cause of reversible inhibition of platelet retention in glass bead columns. *J. Lab. Clin. Med.*, **80**, 603
4. Koepke, J. A., Wu, K. K., Hoak, J. C. and Thompson, J. J. (1975). A comparison of platelet production methods suited for a service orientated blood donor centre. *Transfusion*, **15**, 39

4
Clinical use of Platelet Transfusion in Acute Leukaemia
K. McCredie

INTRODUCTION

Haemorrhage frequently complicates the management of the patient with disseminated malignant disease. It is usually due to thrombocytopenia caused either by bone marrow infiltration with malignant cells or myelosuppression due to therapy[1]. In addition to thrombocytopenia associated with production failure, defects of haemostatic mechanism and qualitative defects of platelets themselves have been described. Disseminated intravascular coagulation associated with rapid platelet consumption, thrombocytopenia, decreased plasma fibrinogen levels and high levels of fibric degradation products has been recognized as causing severe haemorrhage in some patients with malignant disease, particularly acute promyelocytic leukaemia[2]. Although it is important to recognize these other causes of bleeding, thrombocytopenia due to production failure remains the single most important cause of haemorrhage in cancer patients.

Clinical studies have demonstrated the importance of transfusing fresh platelets in preventing and treating haemorrhage due to thrombocytopenia[3]. Early attempts to develop rational platelet transfusion programmes were however hampered by the difficulty of preparing adequate numbers of platelets, their short half life *in vivo*, the failure of storage techniques and the development of resistance in patients receiving multiple transfusions. Most of these problems have been overcome in the last decade.

The modification of plasmapheresis methods has made it possible to obtain large numbers of platelets from individual donors. Using the technique originally described by Yankee, it is possible to obtain plasma, from four units of blood from a single donor containing more than 80% of the platelets separated from the packed red cells (a second spin allows the platelet concentrates to be collected and the platelet poor plasma to be returned to the individual donor)[4]. The limit of plasma that may be removed at pheresis has been defined as being less than 1 litre per week. In fact, a decrease in plasma proteins was only observed in Yankee's series when large quantities of plasma were donated. Donors may be bled weekly for many years without depletion of the serum proteins, and thus plasmapheresis has provided a substantial increase in the number of platelets that can be collected from an individual donor. This is especially relevant to the management of the patient with acute leukaemia or aplastic anaemia since the use of single donor transfusions, particularly from family members considerably reduces the incidence of allo-immunization.

Concentrating platelets from platelet-rich plasma may cause clumping resulting in a reduction in viability after transfusion. However, the identification of the role of adenosine diphosphate and the hydrogen-ion concentration in the platelet-aggregation reaction led to the introduction of the acidification of platelet-rich plasma prior to concentration. As the result of this, platelet increments in recipients of platelets concentrated with acidification are now identical to those obtained with the transfusion of whole platelet-rich plasma. More recently, studies have shown that the use of citrate–phosphate–dextrose as an anticoagulant allows preparation of platelet concentrates with no loss of platelets and with better stability of factor VIII[5]. The preparation of these platelet concentrates has allowed for the administration of larger doses of platelets in shorter periods of time and has diminished the risk of plasma overload in the recipients, particularly in children.

It has been demonstrated that room temperature storage for 24 and even 48 hours under the appropriate conditions is satisfactory for the short-time storage of platelets. However, long term storage decreases the viability in the *in vivo* function of transfused platelets. If the platelets are suspended initially for 1 hour after collection, the clumps seen usually deaggregate and subsequently the platelets can be stored at room temperature (22°C) with agitation and adequate flow of air across for periods of up to 48 hours[6]. Long term storage of platelets, particularly autologous platelets, have been used effectively in replacement in selected patients requiring aggressive platelet support. These platelets have been stored in the presence of cryoprotective agents and it has been demonstrated that platelet viability can be maintained through the freezing and thawing process and that effective control of haemorrhage and elevation of the platelet count can be achieved[7].

CLINICAL EFFECTIVENESS OF PLATELET TRANSFUSION

The rise in the platelet count (increment) in the recipient following transfusion is determined by the number given, their freshness, the method of collection the clinical state of the recipient and his size. The platelet increment is defined as the rise in the platelet count per unit of platelets given (approximately 1×10^{11}) per square metre of the recipient, and is usually between 5 and $10 \times 10^9/l$ 1 hour after transfusion. The median increment calculated from a larger number of series is $10 \times 10^9/l$ and is approximately 25% of the theoretical yield. The increment may be less than expected in the febrile or infected patient who may require transfusion of larger numbers of platelets than if afebrile. Patients actively bleeding require more platelets than patients receiving prophylactic transfusions, and the number of units required cannot be defined numerically but is that needed to stop bleeding. This usually occurs when the platelet count is elevated above $20 \times 10^9/l$.

It has been clearly demonstrated in clinical practice that the frequency and severity of haemorrhage are related to the depth of thrombocytopenia occurring either as the result of marrow infiltration or therapy. Levin *et al.* showed that fatal haemorrhage was only a major risk when the platelet count was below $20 \times 10^9/l$ and was markedly reduced if it was above this level and similarly that all haemorrhage was considerably less common in patients in whom the platelet count was above $50 \times 10^9/l$ than in those in whom it was lower[8].

In a review of the causes of death in patients with cancer, primarily acute leukaemia, it was demonstrated that there was a dramatic reduction in the total number of deaths due to haemorrhage after the introduction of prophylacic platelet transfusions in 1960. The decline in haemorrhage, particularly fatal pulmonary, subarachnoid and intracerebral, was dramatic with an overall reduction of more than 50% of all haemorrhage demonstrated in these patients. It has been noted that severe haemorrhage occurs more frequently as the platelet

41

count approaches the nadir than during the subsequent rise. It is, therefore, generally recommended that prophylactic platelet transfusions be administered to all patients with platelet counts of 20 $\times$ $10^9/l$ or less and that all patients who have evidence of thromboctyopenic bleeding regardless of the platelet count, receive platelet transfusions.

The demonstration of resistance to platelet transfusions has often been associated with transfusion reactions and reduction of platelet survival. The absence of measurable platelet increment and the inability to control haemorrhage usually occurs in patients who have received multiple transfusions. These patients frequently demonstrate antibodies against the HLA histocompatibility antigens and specific platelet antigens. It is possible to obtain satisfactory platelet increments using HLA compatible platelets in selected HLA identical siblings or HLA unrelated compatible donors. It is frequently difficult to find sufficient numbers of unrelated histocompatible identical donors in a random population to provide sufficient HLA compatible long term platelet support. When two HLA antigens or more are shared between the recipient and the donor, adequate transfusion increments can be maintained even in those previously sensitized to HLA antigens and this provides a practical alternative to the use of HLA identical platelets. The average increments corrected as previously described are in the vicinity of 8–12 $\times$ $10^9/l$ one hour after transfusion. Using platelets with one antigen compatible smaller increments are demonstrated in the 5–6 $\times$ $10^9/l$ range; when no antigens are shared between the donor and the recipient, the increments are substantially less[9].

Although the use of HLA compatible platelets may not be necessary in the initial management or short term management of patients with thrombocytopenia, sensitization does occur even in the immunosuppressed patient and it may become necessary to transfuse patients from HLA compatible siblings or non-related donors. The use of these procedures may be particularly important in patients that may require further chemotherapy or bone marrow transplantation.

There are several factors other than the HLA antigens shared which influence the increments seen following platelet transfusion. These include the infection status of the patient, the presence or absence of the spleen and the presence or absence of disseminated intravascular coagulation. Although higher increments are seen in those patients that share HLA antigens, febrile patients show a significant reduction in platelet increments 1 hour after transfusion with median increments in the vicinity of $12 \times 10^9/l$ for the afebrile group compared to $7 \times 10^9/l$ in the febrile group. The presence of a palpable spleen which acts as a reservoir for the platelets has been associated with a substantial reduction in the platelet increments in the compatible groups. In the absence of splenomegaly, the increments achieved were $12 \times 10^9/l$ compared to $4 \times 10^9/l$ in those patients with splenomegaly.

Effective platelet transfusions has also been achieved using platelets stored at room temperature for 24 hours. Studies with such patients have demonstrated that, particularly with HLA compatible patients that fresh platelets and platelets stored for 24 hours give equal increments that survive for equal periods of time within the recipient.

The clinical use of platelet transfusion is now extremely effective, and when used appropriately is rarely unable to prevent or contain haemorrhage in the thrombocytopenic patient at least in the short term. It is, however, essential that those involved in their use do not become complacent, but develop an intelligent approach to thrombocytopenia, bearing in mind the problems of the recipient becoming refractory and the steps which may be taken to prevent it.

References

1. Hersh, E. M., Bodey, G. P., Nies, B. A. and Freireich, E. J. (1965). Causes of death in acute leukaemia. A ten year study of 414 patients. *J. Am. Med. Assoc.*, **193**, 105
2. Whitecar, J. P., Sr. (1971). Disseminated intravascular coagulation in patients with acute leukaemia. *Proc. Am. Assoc. Cancer Res.*, **12**, 46
3. Hirsch, E. O. and Gardner, F. H. (1952). Transfusion of human blood platelets with note on transfusion of granulocytes. *J. Lab. Clin. Med.*, **39**, 556
4. Yankee, R. A., Grumet, F. C. and Rogentine, G. N. (1969). Platelet transfusion therapy. The selection of compatible platelet donors for refractory patients by lymphocyte HLA-typing. *N. Engl. J. Med.*, **281**, 1203
5. Flatow, F. A. and Freireich, E. J. (1966). The increased effectiveness of platelet concentrates prepared in acidified plasma. *Blood*, **27**, 449
6. Murphy, S, and Gardner, F. H. (1969). Platelet preservation. Effect of storage temperature on maintenance of platelet viability-deleterious effect of refrigerated storage. *N. Engl. J. Med.*, **280**, 1094
7. Schiffer, C. A., Aisner, J. and Wiernik, P. H. (1978). Frozen autologous platelet transfusion in patients with leukaemia. *N. Engl. J. Med.*, **299**, 7
8. Levin, R. H., Pert, J. H. and Freireich, E. J. (1965). Response to transfusion of platelets pooled from multiple donors and the effects of various techniques of concentrating platelets. *Transfusion*, **5**, 54

9. Hester, J. P., McCredie, K. B., Lichtiger, H. and Freireich, E. J. (1978). Platelet replacement therapy. A clinical assessment. Presented at the Tenth Annual Red Cross Scientific Symposium, May, 1978.

5
Should Prophylactic Platelets be given to Patients with Acute Leukaemia?

J.M. Ford

Platelet transfusions have been widely available for almost 20 years, but there remain a number of important questions with regard to their optimal clinical application. In this article, I shall address myself to the still highly contentious debate surrounding the usage of prophylactic platelet transfusions. It is probably fair to state that at most centres in the USA where substantial numbers of leukaemic patients are treated a prophylactic transfusion policy is implemented but that this practice is not nearly so widespread in Britain. The discussion will centre on patients with acute leukaemia, primarily because this group currently receive the most active platelet support, but also because such published data that is available, refer almost entirely to leukaemic subjects. I shall begin by outlining the various arguments favouring prophylactic platelets and then give counter-arguments for therapeutic transfusions. The three clinical trials which bear on this subject will be discussed together with some (as yet) unpublished data from this centre. The article will conclude with some recommendations which I feel emerge from the currently available data.

Fundamental to an understanding of the rationale behind prophylactic platelet transfusions are two important clinical observations. In 1962, Gaydos et al. noted in a group of patients with acute leukaemia and co-existent thrombocytopenia that the patients most likely to bleed were those with the lowest platelet counts[1]. In other words, there was a quantitative relationship between the degree of thrombocytopenia and the risk of haemorrhage (Figure 1). Moreover, the relationship held good even when the type of haemorrhage was broken down into three categories of increasing severity (Curves I-III). Most importantly, life-threatening haemorrhage (Curve III) occurred only very infrequently at a platelet count above $10 \times 10^9/l$.

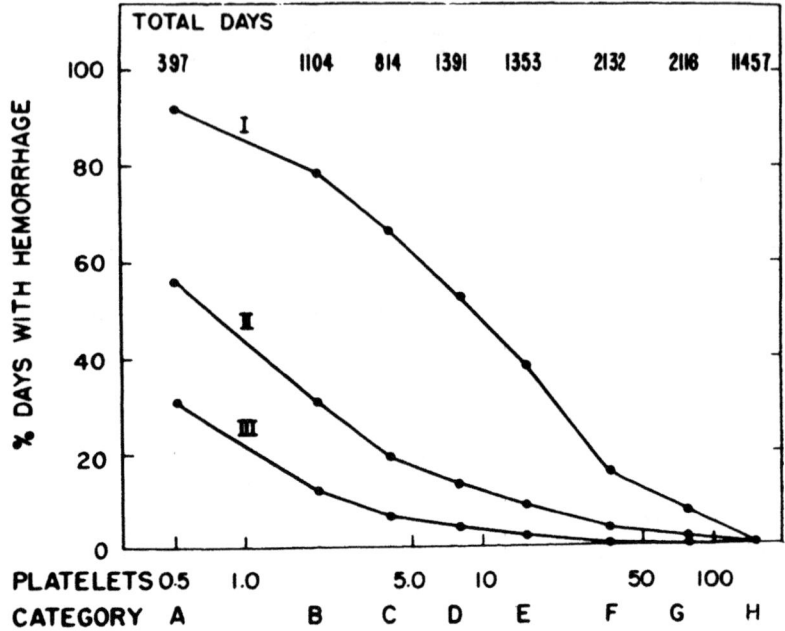

Figure 1 Relation between haemorrhage and platelet count. The percentage of days with haemorrhage in 92 patients is shown for each of 8 platelet categories. Figures across the top are the total number of patient days in each category. Curve I shows data for all haemorrhage manifestations. In Curve II, skin haemorrhage and epistaxis are excluded. Curve III refers only to grossly visible haemorrhage

Harker and Slichter were able to confirm the clinical observations of Gaydos and colleagues by using the bleeding time as a measure of the effectiveness of haemostasis[2]. The striking quantitative relationship between the bleeding time and the level of the platelet count can be seen in Figure 2. Gross prolongation of the bleeding time beyond 25 minutes only occurs when the patient's platelet count is below $20 \times 10^9/l$.

It appears therefore, that there is a critical level for platelets of around $20 \times 10^9/l$ below which haemorrhage is frequent and above which it occurs only rarely. It follows that if the platelet count is maintained above a certain level by transfusion, then the patient should never be at serious risk of sudden massive and even fatal

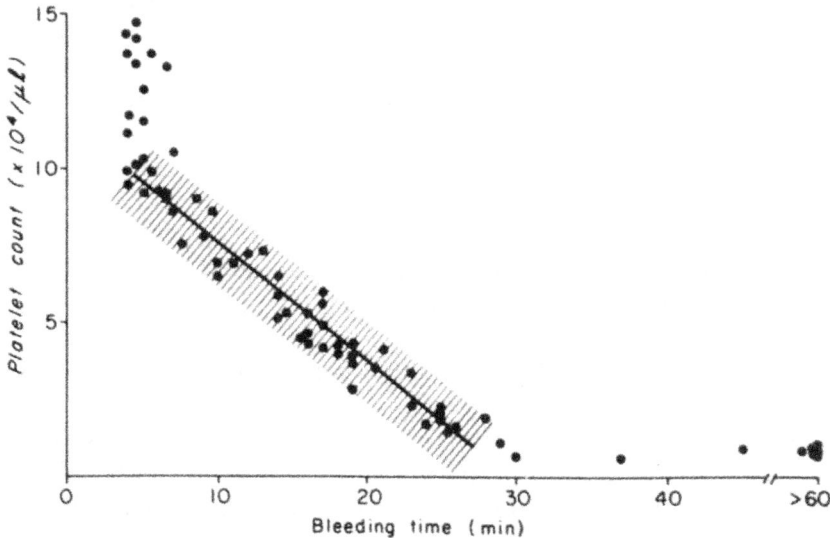

Figure 2 Inverse relation of bleeding time to circulating platelet count in patients with thrombocytopenia

bleeding. In most centres where prophylactic platelets are transfused they are given when the patient's own count falls below 20×10^9 l. With a platelet survival of 9–10 days, this means a transfusion of approximately 4×10^{11} platelets twice weekly for an average sized adult not yet refractory to random donor platelets. The presence of fever, gross splenomegaly or disseminated intravascular coagulation are likely to increase these basic requirements. Most patients will eventually become sensitized to random donor platelets and it is then necessary to use donors who are fully or partially histocompatible with the patient. It is therefore, essential that centres employing a prophylactic platelet support programme, have access to a panel of tissue-typed donors.

The alternative approach, is to transfuse platelets only when the patients show active signs of haemorrhage, i.e. therapeutic platelet transfusions. It has frequently been pointed out that many patients tolerate extremely low platelet counts for long periods of time without showing any signs of bleeding. It may therefore be justifiable to continue to observe such patients because only very occasionally will a fatal bleed occur without any premonitory signs or symptoms. It is argued that, used in this way, fewer platelets will be given with

47

obvious economic implications. In addition, the patients will be exposed to fewer blood products thus reducing (but not eliminating) the likelihood of sensitization.

Any clinical trial investigating the relative efficacy of prophylactic versus therapeutic platelet transfusion therapy should therefore concern itself with three main areas:

1. The death rate in the two groups.
2. The relative numbers of platelet units needed.
3. The relative rates of sensitization.

The three published comparative studies dealing with platelet support will now be discussed.

In 1974, Higby *et al.* reported a study involving 21 periods of marrow aplasia in a group of 18 patients with acute myeloid leukaemia (Table 1)[3]. The subjects were randomized into two groups, the trial patients receiving platelets (approximately 3 units/m^2) twice per week while the controls received the plasma obtained at platelet pheresis to exclude the possibility that some factor other than the platelets was responsible for any benefit observed. In both groups full platelet support was given to any patient who developed signs of haemorrhage.

Table 1

	Patients given platelets	Patients given plasma
No. of aplastic episode	12	9
Mean age	50	57
Haemorrhage absent	7	I
Haemorrhage present (febrile)	5 (4)	8 (6)
Severe haemorrhage present	3 (25%) p 0.05	6 (66%)
Platelet counts		
Average	22 000	17 000
Highest	40 000	41 000
Lowest	2 000	4 000

(Data from Higby *et al*[3])

The study was blind in that the doctors assessing the patients for bleeding did not know whether the patient was receiving platelets or plasma. In the 12 patients given platelets, seven were completely free of haemorrhage whereas in nine controls only one was totally free of bleeding ($p < 0.05$). Severe haemorrhage was present in 25% of the patients given prophylactic platelets, but in 66% of the controls. All patients who bled were febrile at the time of haemorrhage, confirming a previously observed relationship between haemorrhage and fever in thrombocytopenic subjects[4]. There were no deaths in this study and the authors did not compare the number of platelets given to each group. No details of sensitization were reported, although it is clearly crucial to know if the patients who bled despite prophylactic platelets, were refractory to them.

An important point established by Higby et al. was that the dose of platelets transfused was insufficient to elevate the platelet count for a significant portion of the patients' clinical course. Indeed, the mean platelet counts as well as the highest and lowest counts were not significantly different in the two groups, suggesting that bleeding can be prevented even though the platelet count is not held above some arbitrary level.

Murphy et al. studied 90 children with various types of acute leukaemia over a $3\frac{1}{2}$-year period[5]. The prophylactic group received platelets whenever their count fell below $20 \times 10^9/l$, while the patients given therapeutic platelets were transfused in the following circumstances: epistaxis uncontrolled by packing, gross gastrointestinal bleeding, gross haematuria, central nervous system bleeding or any bleeding episode felt to be directly life threatening. The prophylactic group of 39 patients had a mean of 0.9 serious bleeding episodes per patient in comparison to 2.6 bleeds per patient in 51 controls ($p = 0.001$).

The authors were unable to detect a clear difference in sensitization between the two groups. Poor platelet increments following transfusions could usually be attributed to bleeding, infection or splenomegaly – factors known to cause reduced platelet survival[4]. However, they commented that since most of their patients had acute lymphoblastic leukaemia and since all were children, the period of platelet support tended to be much shorter than in an adult patient group with (predominantly) myelogenous leukaemia. In other words, more problems might have been seen if a greater number of transfusions had been given over a longer period of time. No comments were offered on the numbers of platelet transfusions given to the two groups.

Table 2

	Patients given platelets prophylactically	Patients given platelets therapeutically
No. of patients	17	12
No. of courses of chemotherapy	22	17
Mean age	45	44
Bleeding deaths	2	0
Platelet packs given	32	16

(Data from Solomon et al. [6])

A third study by Solomon et al. having the same basic design as the earlier studies appeared in a letter to the *Lancet* (Table 2)[6]. Prophylactic platelets were given to the transfused group when the patient's platelet count fell below $20 \times 10^9/l$. Platelets were again given to controls when active blood loss occurred, but also if a platelet count of $20 \times 10^9/l$ was preceded by a decline of 50% in the platelet count during the preceding 24 hours, a policy which could almost be interpreted as prophylaxis for the controls. All patients were previously untreated adults with myelogenous leukaemia and the two groups were comparable with regard to age and amount of chemotherapy given. In 17 prophylactically transfused patients, there were two bleeding deaths while in the 12 controls, no patient died due to haemorrhage alone. The controls received only half the number of platelets given to the prophylactic group. Not unnaturally, the authors concluded that prophylactic platelets were wasteful of a scarce resource and of no benefit in saving lives.

This statement is difficult to accept for two major reasons. Firstly, the control patients with the most rapidly falling counts received what many investigators would regard as prophylactic platelet support and were, therefore, never at serious risk of haemorrhage. Secondly, (and of greater importance), no details are provided about the degree of sensitization observed during the study. Clearly if the deaths occurred in patients refractory to platelets then any amount of prophylactic support would be ineffectual unless the platelets came from closely matched donors. In the absence of this information, it is difficult to accept the conclusions drawn by Solomon and his co-workers.

A randomized controlled prophylactic granulocyte transfusion trial, the preliminary results of which have already been published[7], was carried out at St Bartholomew's Hospital between 1975 and 1977. The patients were aged between 14 and 59 years and had previously untreated acute myelogenous leukaemia. The granulocytes were obtained from friends and relatives of the patient without regard to HLA matching using a Haemonetics Model 30 and each bag contained a mean of 1.5×10^{10} granulocytes plus 8×10^{11} platelets.

The combined granulocytes and platelets were transfused on alternate days, giving a mean 1-hour platelet increment of approximately $80 \times 10^9/1$ per m². The control patients were not given granulocytes and received platelets from single or pooled donors only if they had clinical signs of bleeding (including skin purpura). Because of the design of this study, it is possible (fortuitously) to analyse the data as a trial of prophylactic versus therapeutic platelet transfusions.

The transfused group comprised 26 patients and there were 23 controls (Table 3). In the transfused patients only one patient had skin bleeding as the sole manifestation of haemorrhage in comparison to five controls. An additional two patients in the transfused group had skin bleeding plus epistaxis while 14 controls had skin haemorrhage plus frank blood loss from a variety of sites. No bleeding was observed in 23 transfused patients, whereas only two controls were free of haemorrhage. The three patients who had bleeding despite transfusion were sensitized to their donors as judged by the absence of a platelet increment and obvious transfusion reactions.

Table 3

	Transfused	Controls
No. of patients	26	23
Patients with skin haemorrhage alone	1	5
Patients with skin haemorrhage plus other sites of blood loss	2	14
Patients with no haemorrhage	23	2
Haemorrhagic deaths	0	1

St Barthomomew's Hospital data

(Data from Higby et al.)[4]

There were no deaths due to haemorrhage in the transfused patients, although one patient died of uncertain cause – a post mortem having been refused on religious grounds. A 57-year-old female control died secondary to a massive sub-mucosal bleed of the small intestine during a period when she was markedly febrile.

Clearly, it would not be profitable to analyse this study in terms of numbers of platelets transfused, since many more platelets were given to the transfused group than would ordinarily be scheduled in a formal prophylactic platelet trial. However, of central importance is the finding that a control patient died unexpectedly of haemorrhage at a time when she was febrile. In other words, a patient died from a preventable complication before she had had an adequate trial of chemotherapy.

From the data available, there seems little doubt that maintaining the patient's platelet count above a level of approximately $20 \times 10^9/l$ will greatly reduce the incidence of haemorrhage. Conversely, similar patients not given platelet transfusions will have significantly more serious bleeding episodes. The data of Higby and colleagues is of interest since it suggests that the intregrity of the blood vessels can be preserved without necessarily giving sufficient platelets to raise the circulating platelet count by any significant degree. Profuse bleeding must be a terrifying experience for these unfortunate patients. Indeed, it is difficult to imagine a more graphic demonstration to the patient of the seriousness of his condition than a sudden unexpected copious haemorrhage. Somehow, infective episodes – although of much greater concern to the attending medical staff – are much less alarming to the patient.

It seems likely that this policy will also save the lives of a small proportion of cases. Although some patients tolerate very low platelet counts without bleeding and the majority of the remainder will have a minor warning bleed before having life-threatening haemorrhage, the occasional patient will die as a result of sudden, massive bleeding into a critical part of the body. In our study, we lost a patient in precisely this fashion following a bleed into the gut wall, though it is likely that central nervous system haemorrhage constitutes the greatest threat. A large scale controlled trial involving several hundred patients would be required to confirm this thesis, because by extrapolation from our data, it would appear that the mortality rate due to bleeding in patients given therapeutic platelets is of the order of 5%.

Much greater uncertainty surrounds the rate of sensitization resulting from prophylactic platelet support and studies carried out to date shed little light on this aspect. It seems likely that more platelets are transfused when given prophylactically and that the increased numbers of transfusions means that more patients are likely to become sensitized. It is for this reason that the data of Higby *et al.* is of such interest. However, great progress is being made in the use of HLA-matched platelets[8], selectively HLA mis-matched platelets[9] and autologous frozen platelets[10] and hence sensitized patients are becoming increasingly easy to support.

In summary, despite the increased cost, it seems reasonable to recommend that prophylactic platelet transfusions be given to patients with acute leukaemia because of the great reduction in morbidity due to haemorrhage and a probable small reduction in deaths due to bleeding. Platelets should be given when the patient's count is less than $20 \times 10^9/l$ especially in the presence of fever or if the count is falling due to uncontrolled disease or recent chemotherapy. Although platelet counts of less than $10 \times 10^9/l$ usually indicate the need for support, counts of between 10–$20 \times 10^9/l$ can sometimes be observed without any action being taken. For instance, platelet transfusions are not indicated in afebrile patients approaching the end of predictable platelet nadirs (as during consolidation chemotherapy) or if a recent marrow shows early megakaryocyte regeneration. It cannot be emphasized too strongly that, in order to reduce or delay both the incidence and degree of sensitization, prophylactic platelets should be ordered only after thoughtful consideration of the patient's clinical condition and of the proximity of recent myelosuppressive chemotherapy.

References

1. Gaydos, L. A., Freireich, E. J. and Mantel, N. (1962). The quantitative relation between platelet count and haemorrhage in patients with acute leukaemia. *N. Engl. J. Med.*, **266**, 905
2. Harker, L. A. and Slichter, S. J. (1972). The bleeding time as a screening test for evaluation of platelet function. *N. Engl. J. Med.*, **287**, 155
3. Higby, D. J., Cohen, E., Holland, J. F. and Sinks, L. (1974). The prophylactic treatment of thrombocytopenic leukaemic patients with platelets: a double blind study. *Transfusion*, **14**, 440
4. Alvarado, J., Djerassi, I. and Farber, S. (1965). Transfusion of fresh concentrated platelets to children with acute leukaemia. *J. Paediatr.*, **67**, 13
5. Murphy, S., Koch, P. A. and Evans, A. E. (1976). Randomized trial of prophylactic versus therapeutic platelet transfusion in childhood acute leukaemia. *Clin. Res.*, **3**, 379 A (abstract)

6. Solomon, J., Bolenkamp, T., Fahey, J. L., Chillar, R. K. and Beutler, E. (1978). Platelet prophylaxis in acute non-lymphoblastic leukaemia. *Lancet*, **1**, 267

7. Ford, J. M. and Cullen, M. H. (1977). Prophylactic granulocyte transfusions. *Exp. Haematol.*, **5**, (Suppl 1), 65

8. Yankee, R. A., Graff, K. S., Dowling, R. and Henderson, E. S. (1973). Selection of unrelated compatible platelet donors by lymphocyte HLA-matching. *N. Engl. J. Med.*, **288**, 760

9. Duquesnoy, R. J., Filip, D. J., Rodey, G. E., Rimm, A. A. and Aster, R. H. (1977). Successful transfusion of platelets 'mismatched' for HLA antigens to alloimmunized thrombocytopenic patients. *Am. J. Haematol.*, **2**, 219

10. Schiffer, C. A., Aisner, J. and Wiernick, P. H. (1978). Frozen autologous platelet transfusion for patients with leukaemia. *N. Engl. J. Med.*, **299**, 7

Index